# Lyme Disease Explained

Transmission, Diagnosis, Symptoms, Treatment, Prognosis, Infectious Diseases, Vaccines, History, Myths, and More!

By Frederick Earlstein

# Foreword

Lyme disease is fast becoming a growing concern in the United States and around the world. It is estimated that about 300,000 people in the U.S. get Lyme disease each year, according to the CDC. The World Health Organization estimates about 35,000 yearly cases in Europe, and another 3,500 or so in Asia. And because of various factors such as undiagnosed and misdiagnosed cases, the numbers may actually be a lot higher.

These numbers are expected to grow at double-digit rates in the next couple of years - mainly because of the growing population of infected ticks, and the loss of their natural habitats which sees them moving closer to human-populated areas. This is an alarming statistic to look at - especially since we still do not know enough about this disease to identify and treat it successfully.

But as with any disease, prevention is always better than any cure, and probably the best way of combating this disease, or at least minimizing the incidence of infections - is by spreading awareness about how it is transmitted and how risks of infection can be minimized or avoided. This book aims to assist in this venture by compiling many of the current news, data and facts about Lyme disease for the education and information of the reading public.

# Table of Contents

# Introduction

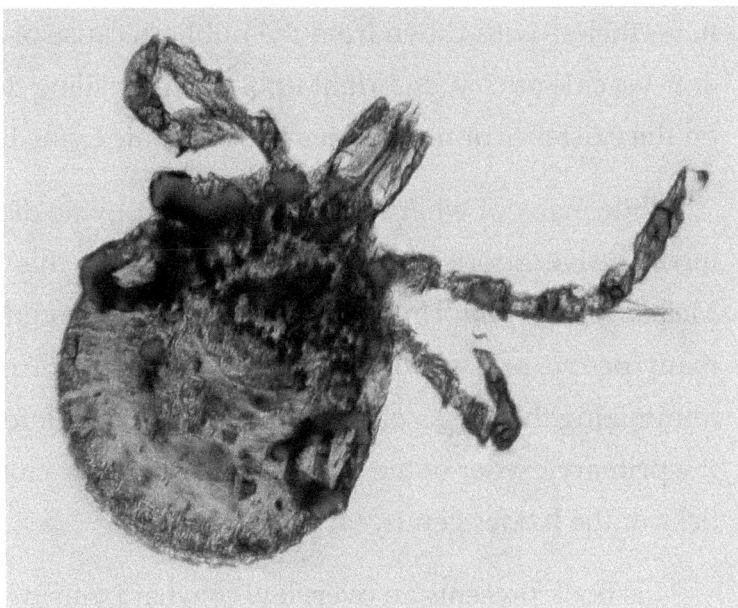

Lyme disease is a difficult condition to pin down - and the elusiveness of this disease has characterized its recent history - from its identification as a distinct infection, to the current struggles at diagnosis and treatments. Experts are not even able to definitively state that the bacteria has been effectively eliminated from the system of a person who has undergone the recommended antibiotic treatments. And controversy of one sort or another has certainly dogged

Lyme disease - from whispers of its being an accidental outbreak of a government laboratory experiments with biological weapons, to the effective vaccine that was nevertheless withdrawn from the public because of a huge anti-vaccine outcry, and right up to the prevailing debates on the existence or non-existence of Chronic Lyme Disease.

While many of what we do know about Lyme disease is inconclusive, efforts are being made to remedy this. Meanwhile, the information that we do have should enable many people to avoid being infected in the first place by minimizing their risks of being bitten and being infected by the primary carrier of the Lyme disease bacteria - infected ticks of the Ixodes genus.

This book presents an overview of what Lyme disease is, how it is transmitted, and how it can be prevented. The primary signs and symptoms are also described to enable people to recognize the possibility of an infection at the earliest opportunity.

Hopefully, this will encourage people to seek medical and professional assistance as soon as possible in order to prevent the disease from spreading, in order to give people the best chance for a full recovery. For those in the later stages of Lyme disease, we have also provided an overview of some of the alternative therapies or holistic remedies that you could explore as you cope with the symptoms of this disease.

Below you will find a glossary of some of the important terms and vocabulary related to Lyme disease.

## *Important Terms to Know*

**Antibiotic** - Drugs used to treat bacterial infections.

**Antibody** - A specialized immune protein produced or triggered by the introduction of an antigen into the body, and which possesses the ability to combat the very antigen that triggered its production in the first place.

**Arthritis** - General name for any type of joint inflammation, though it often refers to age-related osteoarthritis

**Bacterial diseases** - Diseases caused by bacterial infection.

**Bell's Palsy** - A primarily temporary facial nerve disorder where part or the entire face suddenly becomes paralysed.

**Borrelia** - A group of bacteria with helical spirochetes, named after Amedee Borrel, a French bacteriologist.

**Borreliosis** - An infectious bacterial disorder transmitted by ticks.

**Chronic** - Lasting a long time.

**Chronic Fatigue Syndrome** - Severe chronic fatigue disorder that often follows an infection.

**ELISA** - Enzyme-linked immunosorbent assay. This is a first stage serology test to detect levels of Lyme disease antibodies.

**Erythema Migrans** - A bull's eye rash that often appears during the first stage of Lyme disease

**Fibromyalgia** - A condition affecting the musclse and/or joints, which is usually difficult to diagnose.

**Juvenile Rheumatoid Arthritis** - Chronic arthritis taht affects children and teens.

**Lesion** - An area of abnormal tissue change.

**Lyme disease** - An infectious disease caused by tick-borne bacteria of the Borrelia genus.

**Meningitis** - A dangerous infection of the membranes that surround the brain.

**Multiple Sclerosis** - An autoimmune condition affecting the spinal nerves.

**Prognosis** - The probable outcome or course of a disease.

**Rash** - General term for skin inflammations.

**Residual** - Something has been left behind.

**Spirochete** - Microscopic bacterial organism of the Spirochaeta family. They have a worm-like, spiral-shaped form.

# Chapter One: What is Lyme Disease?

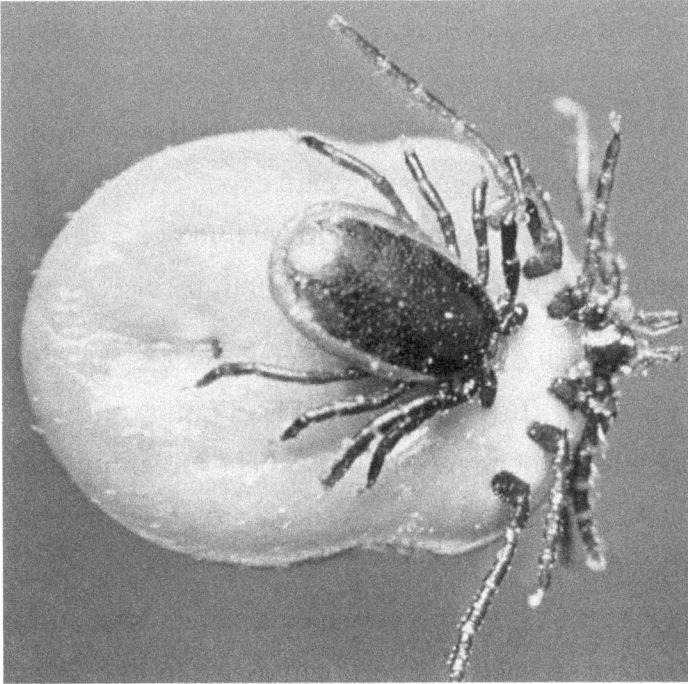

Lyme disease, sometimes also known as Lyme borreliosis, is an infectious disease caused by the bacteria Borrelia burgdorferi. It is transmitted through the bite of infected ticks of the genus Ixodes. The World Health Organization classifies Lyme disease as an infectious or parasitic disease.

This bacterial infection can affect people of all ages, and cases of Lyme disease have been found in every continent except Antarctica. The prevalence rate is pretty high, and it is estimated that at least 300,000 people are diagnosed with Lyme disease every year in the United States, and that there are about 2,000 to 3,000 new cases each year in England and Wales. But these numbers are expected to be much higher because of the number of cases which go undiagnosed, or which are misdiagnosed as something else.

In fact, if detected early, Lyme disease can often be treated effectively. But diagnosing it is not quite so simple. It has sometimes been referred to as "The Great Imitator" because its symptoms are often so similar to many other diseases such as chronic fatigue syndrome, multiple sclerosis, fibromyalgia, and some psychiatric illnesses such as depression. Misdiagnosis can delay appropriate treatment, in which case a person infected with this disease has a higher risk of developing severe and long-lasting symptoms.

Early detection is, therefore, crucial, and information awareness even more so. This book therefore aims to provide you with some of the basic information you will need in identifying cases of Lyme disease, diagnosis, tips for prevention, and treatment.

## History of Lyme Disease

The peculiar name of Lyme Disease derives from a place - Lyme, Connecticut, where a mysterious illness took hold of a group of children and some adults sometime in the early 1970s. What interested researchers in this event was when two of the mothers of these children alerted the state health department to the fact that all of these kids were diagnosed with juvenile rheumatoid arthritis.

A doctor at Yale University named Allen Steere investigated the occurrence, and in 1977, he published a paper in the medical journal *Arthritis and Rheumatism* identifying a new disease which he called Lyme arthritis, which was transmitted by ticks. Soon afterwards, it became known as Lyme disease. The specific cause, however, was as yet unidentified.

In the 1980s, Willy Burgdorfer, a scientist who was then studying Rocky Mountain Spotted Fever began to study Lyme disease. Both these diseases were caused by tick bites, and soon he found the connection. The spirochete bacterium was identified as the causative agent of Lyme disease, and which were transmitted through tick bites, or via the tick's salivary glands. In 1982, the spirochete was named Borrelia burgdorferi in honor of Dr. Burgdorfer's discovery.

For a time, conspiracy theorists have postulated that the sudden emergence of Lyme disease was due to an accidental release of infected ticks from Plum Island - located off the coast of Long Island, New York, and just a few miles off the coast of Lyme, Connecticut. This theory became popular after the publication of Michael C. Carroll's book, *Lab 257: The Disturbing Story of the Government's Secret Plum Island Germ Laboratory*. Essentially, Plum Island was a military base-turned-government animal disease center, and now being operated by the Department of Homeland Security, whose research efforts allegedly revolve around agricultural bioterrorism, particularly the development of various diseases intended as biological weapons. Carroll's book cites experiments that use ticks as disease carriers for germ warfare.

More recent discoveries, however, have supplied scientists with evidence that Lyme Disease is a lot older than Plum Island - and a 5,300 year old mummy discovered along the Austria-Italy border in 1991, thereafter named Ötzi the Iceman, was believed to have suffered from Lyme disease. In fact, genetic analysis has shown that the bacteria Borrelia burgdorferi is quite ancient, and of European origin. Several early accounts of the skin manifestations of what is now known as Lyme disease have been documented in some European countries such as Scotland, Germany, France, and Sweden.

Though it does seem that genetic variations may have existed across the present-day United States before European settlement. As settlers moved west across the United States, clearing forests in their wake, the populations of deer and white-footed mice dwindled. These two were some of the main hosts for the black-legged ticks, and where they survived - mainly in the Northeast and the Midwest, the tick parasites also survived, traveling to new habitat as their hosts moved into regenerated forests in the abandoned farm fields in New England in the mid-19th century. The outward spread of Lyme disease from these areas are believed to have been borne by migratory birds, as they now expand their ranges north.

Some have identified other various factors which may have resulted in the more recent spread of this disease: global warming is a possible link, but mainly urbanization and the spread of suburban neighborhoods, deforestation, and increased contact between humans and tick-dense areas, together with the reduced population of the primary hosts of ticks such as small rodents, mice, and chipmunks, may have been instrumental in the spread of Lyme disease among human populations.

Since then, the spread of Lyme disease has grown exponentially all over the world, occurring regularly in the temperate regions of the Northern Hemisphere. It has been included as one of the top ten notifiable diseases by the CDC (Centers for Disease Control and Prevention).

## Myths About Lyme Disease

Proper education and accurate information is always one of the best ways we have to counteract any disease or illness - and Lyme disease is no exception. But perhaps because the identification of this disease has been fairly recent - or because of its similarity to many other diseases, certain myths have grown around this fast-growing epidemic. Here are some of the major misconceptions that people have about Lyme disease:

- *That Lyme disease always comes with a bull's eye rash.* While some instances of Lyme disease does carry the distinctive bully's eye rash, this is not always true. In fact, it is estimated that only less than 50%

of patients diagnosed with Lyme disease have this characteristic rash, and the rest never do. Many of the symptoms are far less distinct, such as a simple rash, a stiff neck, or mild flu-like symptoms.

- *That Lyme disease is isolated to certain areas or regions, such as the East Coast of the United States, Europe, or even primarily in rural areas.* This is a dangerous misconception, since it causes people to assume that they are safe. But the thing to remember is that Lyme disease is primarily transmitted by ticks, and ticks can survive on any number of hosts, many of which can cross geographical boundaries and regions such as birds, mice, chipmunks, squirrels, deer, and even dogs and cats. Lyme disease is a global problem, and cases of it have been reported in most parts of the United States, and it has also been found to be endemic to Asia, parts of Europe, Australia, Canada, and even in the Amazon region of Brazil.

- *That a negative blood test means you don't have Lyme disease.* The fact of it is that the current two-tiered blood test for Lyme disease does not test for the presence or absence of the bacteria itself. What it measures are your body's antibodies against the bacteria Borrelia burgdorferi. So if your antibodies are not high enough to be detected, your results can show up as a false negative, especially in the early stages of this disease. This test alone can miss up to 60% of acute cases of Lyme, and is not considered definitive basis for a diagnosis.

- *You can't get Lyme disease in the winter, or that ticks die in winter.* Deer ticks can survive in very cold climates, and they live for an average of two years. For a tick to start dying, temperatures have to drop to below 10 degrees Fahrenheit, which is not true in many regions, despite the winter season, and particularly now because of climate change.

- *All ticks carry Borrelia burgdorferi, or that all tick bites can result in Lyme disease.* Not all ticks carry the bacteria Borrelia burgdorferi, therefore not all ticks can transmit Lyme disease. In fact, even a bite from an infected tick does not necessarily result in an infection. According to the CDC, a tick must be attached for 36 to 48 hours before the Lyme bacterium can be transmitted, so an immediate removal of the tick is best. Of course, not all tick bites are noticeable, and because of the numbing agent in their saliva, you probably won't even realize that they are feeding on you.

- *A tick is best removed using Methylated Spirits, Vaseline, Ether, by burning them with a match, or suffocating them with nail polish, gasoline, or petroleum jelly.* The best option you have to removing a tick is actually a lot simpler: gently pull the tick away from the skin, making sure that the tick's mouth parts are also removed.

- *That Doxycycline can prevent you from contracting Lyme disease, or that Doxycycline cures Lyme quickly.* While some cases of Lyme disease can be cured quickly with *tetracycline* antibiotics such as *doxycycline* or other antibiotics such as *penicillin* or *cephalosporin,* provided the condition was diagnosed and treated within two to four weeks from the transmission of the disease, not everybody is always fortunate. Studies have found that about 25% of patients still exhibit symptoms even after treatment. It can take a long time before a patient feels completely well. Some have referred to this as chronic Lyme disease, though it bears stressing that there is an ongoing controversy about the existence of Chronic Lyme disease in the first place, as opposed to what the CDC has referred to as post-treatment Lyme disease syndrome (PTLDS), which they claim are merely lingering symptoms after after antibiotic treatments. And repeated cases of Lyme disease may simply be a reinfection, not a relapse.

# Chapter Two: Ticks of the Ixodes Genus and the Family Ixodidae

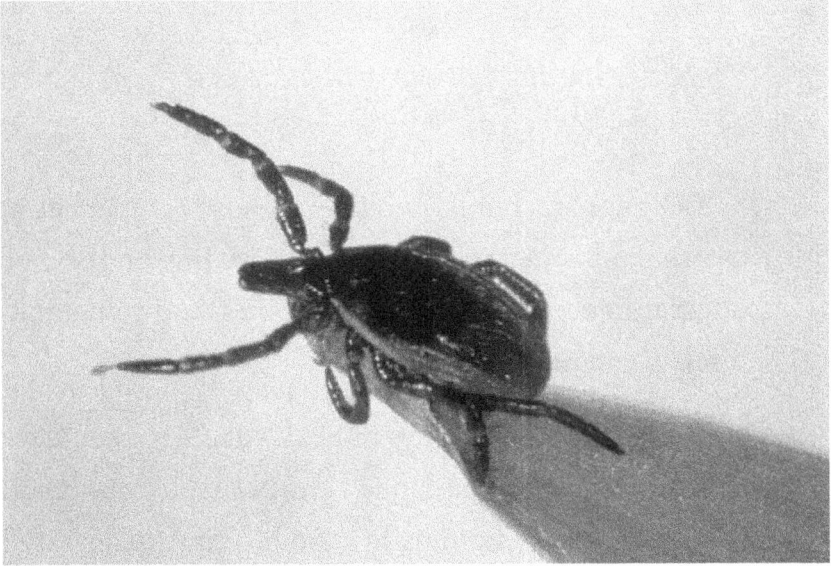

Not all ticks are carriers of the Borrelia burgdorferi bacteria, simply because not all ticks *can* be carriers.  So one of the best ways of counteracting or preventing Lyme disease is getting to know the primary transmitter of this disease.  This chapter contains some basic information on what ticks are carriers, how to recognize them, where they can be found, and how they act as vectors for diseases among both humans and animals.  We will also cover how

to avoid getting bitten by a tick, and what to do if you get
bitten.

## *What are the ticks of the genus Ixodes?*

Ticks are arachnids, and they are also ectoparasites, or
external parasites, and they live by feeding on the blood of
other animals such as mammals, birds, and sometimes
reptiles and amphibians.

There are three families of ticks - the Nuttaliellidae, the
Argasidae, and the Ixodidae. The Nuttaliellidae are a single
species of tick found mostly in Southern Africa, and differ
strongly in appearance and structure from the other two.
The following table, on the other hand, helps to illustrate the
difference between the other two families of ticks:

| Ixodidae | Argasidae |
|---|---|
| Considered the "hard ticks;" they have a hard shield or a scutum | Have no scutum and are soft-bodied |
| Have a prominent capitulum (head) that | The capitulum is concealed beneath the |

| | |
|---|---|
| projects forward from the body | body |
| bite is painless and goes generally unnoticed | bite is painful |
| will remain in place on the host for a long time | will gorge within minutes and will not stay with the host for a long time |
| Have no fixed dwelling place, other than on the host | live in sand or crevices and emerge only to feed |
| Feeds on mammals, birds, and sometimes reptiles and amphibians | Feeds primarily on birds, but will also sometimes attack mammals |

There are over 700 species of Ixodidae ticks, but one genus - the Ixodes, are the primary transmitters of the Borrelia burgdorferi bacterium which is the cause of Lyme disease.  There are four recognized primary vectors of Lyme disease in the world, and these include:

- the Ixodes scapularis (deer tick) in North America and the East Coast
- the Ixodes ricinus in Europe
- the Ixodes persulcatus in China and Asia

- the Ixodes pacificus on the West Coast.

## *How ticks transmit diseases*

You might think that a hard-bodied tick that feeds for a long time on a host should be easy to spot, and therefore easy to get rid of. But it isn't that simple. For one thing, the Ixodidae tick secretes a local anesthetic that prevent the host from feeling any itch or pain from its bite, so chances are that you might not even realize that you have been bitten. And for another, it is estimated that most infections are caused by bites from nymphs - or ticks in the nymphal stage - which are smaller (about the size of a poppy seed), and therefore more difficult to detect. Though it bears stressing that both infected nymphs and infected adults are capable of transmitting the disease to the new host.

It is interesting to note that while humans contract Lyme disease primarily from tick bites - ticks are not the main source of the Borrelia burgdorferi bacteria. Indeed, this is an infectious disease mostly found among animals such as deer, small mammals, and birds, and are transmitted to humans in a process called zoonosis, through tick bites.

Ticks go through three primary stages of development: from a larva, to a nymph, and then to an adult. As they move from one stage to another, they also move among three different hosts. After feeding from one host, they detach and molt, eventually feeding on progressively larger hosts as they molt again and grow to become adults. In each case, they will need to feed on blood to survive and to move from one life stage to another.

The primary diet of ticks is blood, and this is known as hematophagy. They contract the Borrelia burgdorferi bacteria if they feed on infected animals such as deer, rodents or birds. It then carries the bacteria in its belly or midgut, where it is retained as it moves through its molting stage and until it attaches itself to a new host. Once it starts feeding again, the bacteria will migrate from the midgut to its salivary glands, where it will then be injected into the new host's bloodstream.

It does take time for the bacteria to move into the host's bloodstream, but because of the size of the nymphal ticks, and the anesthetic they secrete, a person is not likely to notice them until they have grown larger in size - by which time the probability of the disease having been transmitted is greater.

## How to Avoid Tick Bites

It seems apparent that one of the best ways we have of avoiding contracting Lyme disease in the first place is to minimize the risk of getting bitten by ticks. This is particularly important for those who spend much of their time in the outdoors, in woods, near rivers, or other places where there is a population of small animals. Ticks also thrive in moist and humid environments such as grassy or woody areas. Campers, hikers and even gardeners should be doubly careful.

The following are some tips you can follow to avoid getting bitten by ticks:

- Check for ticks immediately after you have spent time outdoors. Showering immediately, or within two hours after coming indoors, can wash off any unattached ticks, is a good time to check for ticks, and can greatly reduce your risk of getting Lyme disease. Pay particular attention to your scalp, underarms, inside the belly button, in and around the ears, the backs of the knees, around the waist, or between your legs and the groin area.

- Stay on trails or paths as much as possible, and stay out of tall grasses or brush
- Reduce the amount of exposed skin, for instance by tucking in your pants into your socks
- Use an insect repellant that contains 20-30% DEET on any exposed skin and clothing. A 20% or more DEET can protect up to several hours. Always remember to follow product instructions when applying repellant on skin.
- Treat your clothing and footwear with permethrin-based repellant, which can kill ticks. Take note that this kind of repellant can still be effective even after several washings.
- If you have been bitten by a tick, or been in the outdoors, and develop a fever and a rash a few weeks later, see a doctor immediately. Remember that the incubation period for tick-born diseases is 8-14 days.
- If you have any dogs or cats, provide them with a tick collar or monthly treatments so that they will not carry ticks home with them.
- Examine your clothes, your gear, and your pets for the possible presence of ticks.

- Tumble-dry your clothes in a dryer set at high heat
  for 10 minutes to kill ticks. If the clothes are damp,
  increase the time. If you need to wash your clothes
  first, use hot water. If this is not possible, tumble
  dry at low heat for 70 minutes or at high heat for 40
  minutes. In all instances, the clothes should be
  warm and completely dry.
- Reduce the possibility of the presence of ticks in
  your home by discouraging the presence of small
  animals, and by removing possible tick habitats
  such as leaf piles, shrubs and groundcover. Any
  outdoor equipment or furniture should be kept in
  the sun and away from the shade.
- If you do find a tick, remove it properly (see below)

## *How to Properly Remove a Tick*

It is important not to panic if you should find a tick
attached to the skin. Some people may have an immediate
tendency to remove the tick immediately by picking it off
using tweezers of one's fingers, but doing so recklessly may
actually do more harm than good. Doing so may cause you
to squeeze the tick so that it regurgitates its fluids into your

bloodstream. Jerking or twisting the tick might also cause
you to leave behind some of its mouth parts in your skin.

On the other hand, you will also need to act quickly.
Remember that the goal is to remove the tick as quickly as
possible to reduce the risk of infection. Remedies such as
using nail polish, a the heat from a lit match, or petroleum
jelly is, therefore, discouraged, as waiting for the tick to
detach in the meantime only prolongs the tick's contact and
thus increases the risk of infection.

The following are steps in the proper removal of a tick:

1. Use a fine-tipped tweezer to grasp the tick as close
   to the skin as possible.
2. Remove it by applying a steady, upward force,
   being careful not to squeeze the tick, and to avoid
   leaving behind some of its mouth parts embedded
   in the  skin. If this does happen, remove the mouth
   parts with the tweezers.
3. Disinfect the bite area thoroughly, using alcohol,
   iodine scrub, or soap and water.
4. Submerge the tick in alcohol and place it in a
   sealed bag or container. Note carefully the details
   of where and when the bite occurred. You can

either dispose of the tick by wrapping it tightly in tape and flushing it down the toilet, or you can store the tick for later identification. Testing a tick for Lyme disease is usually not helpful or even conclusive.

5. If the tick's head and mouthparts were left in the skin, a punch biopsy may be necessary to remove any parts that were left behind.

# Chapter Three: Signs and Symptoms and the Stages of Lyme Disease

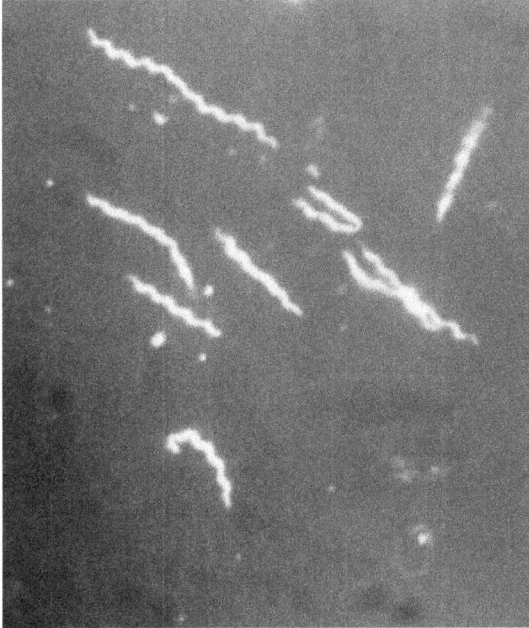

Lyme disease is an infection caused by the Borrelia burgdorferi bacterium. In this chapter we take a closer look at this invading microogranism and the effects of its invasion into a person's body. The signs and symptoms and their severity which a person will experience depends on the dissemination of the infection in a person's body, which are classified according to three different stages.

It bears stressing that different strains of the Borrelia
bacteria cause Lyme disease in different areas or regions in
the world. Borrelia burgdorferi is the most common strain
found in the United States, though it is by no means
exclusive.

## *Lyme Disease Pathology*

The spirochete Borrelia burgdorferi, which are spirally-
shaped bacteria, is transmitted into a person's skin via the
tick's saliva. This saliva has certain components which
disrupt the body's normal immune response, thereby also
providing protection to the infectious bacteria, allowing
them to settle themselves in the local area.

As the spirochetes multiply, they spread outwards over
the skin, causing the characteristic bull's eye rash, also called
erythema migrans - though again not everybody who gets
Lyme disease will manifest this characteristic rash. In the
following days and weeks, they will slowly enter the
bloodstream, where they can then gain access to the rest of
the body's tissues, via the circulatory system. As the bacteria
spreads, so do the symptoms. The incubation period, or the

time from infection to the time when the symptoms appear,
is variable - sometimes a few days, or as long as several
months or even years.  In general however, it takes about
one to two weeks before symptoms manifest.

Many of the symptoms that a person manifests actually
stem from the responses of their immune system to the
foreign bacteria in each localized area.  The difficulty is that
the Borrelia burgdorferi bacteria is pretty adept at hiding
itself.

When the body detects a foreign invader, the immune
system mounts certain defenses, including inflammatory
responses and the production of neutrophils, which aid the
body in fighting infection.  But even as body mounts its
defenses, there is never enough production of neutrophils -
mainly because they cannot find or detect the foreign
invader.

The Borrelia burgdorferi bacteria makes use of the protein
plasmin from the tick's saliva to hide from the immune
system, while at the same time reducing its expression of
surface protein - which are what are usually targeted by
neutrophils.  It might also be possible that the Borrelia
burgdorferi avoids detection by mimicking some of the

body's proteins because of similar epitopes. They are thus
perceived as non-threatening, or are even accepted by the
body as its own. So while the body sets itself up to defend
itself, it does not produce enough antibodies or neutrophils
to effectively combat the foreign invader. Meanwhile, the
bacteria spreads and thrives, surpassing and, in the process,
interfering with the immune system.

While proving ineffective agains the invading bacteria,
the body's lengthy and damaging immunological response
to the presence of a foreign invader are largely what cause
many of the symptoms of Lyme disease. The bacteria
imitates normal body cells, confusing a person's immune
system, which can then attack ordinary body tissues. When
the body starts producing antibodies against its own cells, it
throws the immune system completely out of balance,
possibly causing autoimmune conditions. The chronic
nature of Lyme disease can often be traced to this resulting
disorder within the immune system, which continues even
when the Borrelia bacteria has already been removed.

## The Three Stages of Lyme Disease

Because of the pervasiveness of the bacteria Borrelia
burgdorferi, it can have a multisystem effect, and multiple
organs and systems in the body can be affected. The
symptoms are highly variable, and not everyone can
experience all the identified symptoms of Lyme disease.
Many of these signs and symptoms are similar to those
experienced with other diseases, which often lead to
misdiagnosis. For this reason, and perhaps due to the
adaptive nature of the bacteria Borrelia burgdorferi itself in
hiding within a person's system, Lyme disease has
sometimes been referred to as "The Great Imitator."

The progress of Lyme disease is based on the spread of
the bacteria within a person's system, and the level of
inflammation and the resulting tissue damage. As the
disease advances, more bodily systems become affected, and
the symptoms grow more severe.

### Stage 1: Early Localized
In the early localized stage, Lyme disease visibly affects
the skin. Erythma migrans (EM) is one of the best clinical

indicators, though this only occurs in about 50% of those
who are infected. EM starts as a red papule at the site of the
tick bite, appearing within 3 to 32 days after the bite. When
the infection spreads, the reddish area also expands, creating
a larger reddish ring around the center, and a clear area in
between - resembling a bull's eye. This may be hot to the
touch, or warm, but is generally painless. The inner rash
grows a darker red, and becomes indurated - or thicker and
firmer to the touch.

In other cases, the EM appears as a simple red lesion
without the bull's eye appearance, and there are those who
will not develop any sort of rash at all. These usually fades
or disappears within the next 3 to 4 weeks.

A person may also develop other, flu-like symptoms such
as headaches, muscle soreness, malaise, fatigue, chills, stiff
neck, fever, myalgias, and arthralgias. When a person
develops these flu-like symptoms, without having shown
signs of EM or a rash, there is a great possibility of
misdiagnosis. But while the symptoms may be intermittent,
malaise and fatigue may still linger for several weeks.

Other possible symptoms, though less common, include backacke, nausea, vomiting, sore throat, lymphadenopathy, and splenomegaly.

### Stage 2: Early Disseminated

As the infection spreads, EM, or smaller and secondary lesions may appear in other locations other than the original site of the tick bite, but without the inundurated centers. In Europe, some patients also develop borrelial lymphocytoma, which is a purplish lump that can develop either on the ear lobe, nipple, or the scrotum. A person may also experience some brief arthritis attacks, and migratory pain in the joints.

Some 15% of patients also develop certain neurological problems, such as lymphocitic meningitis, Bell palsy, cranial neuritis, radicoloneuritis, meningoencephalitis, and neuroborreliosis. Cardiac problems may also manifest in the form of atrioventricular block, myopericarditis with chest pain, pancarditis, and cardiomegaly.

Secondary symptoms that may arise from the above conditions can include severe headaches, neck stiffness, sensitivity to light, sleep disturbances, memory loss, mood changes, abnormal heart rhythm, malaise and fatigue,

abnormal skin sensations, and an inflammation of the spinal
cord's nerve roots which can cause shooting pains.


### Stage 3: Late Disseminated

The late stages of Lyme disease can manifest some
months to years after the initial infection. During this stage,
the infection has spread all throughout a person's body, and
they may develop the following symptoms:

- Prolonged arthritis attacks or chronic arthritis
- Intermittent swelling and pain in large joints,
  especially the knees
- chronic CNS abnormalities, such as
  encephalopathy or polyneuropathy
- leukoencephalitis
- malaise
- fatigue
- low-grade fever
- antibiotic-sensitive skin lesions
- mood, memory and sleep disorders such as
  insomnia
- shooting pains, numbness, and tingling in the
  hands or feet

- cognitive difficulties such as brain fog
- migraines
- balance problems and vertigo
- facial palsy
- bladder problems
- back pain
- dementia
- transverse myelitis

In extreme cases, there may be permanent impairment of motor or sensory function of the lower extremities. Arthritis caused by Lyme disease usually affects the knees, though it can also occur in other joints. The knees will be swollen, hot, and sometimes painful. Baker's cysts may also form and rupture.

# Chapter Four: Diagnosing Lyme Disease

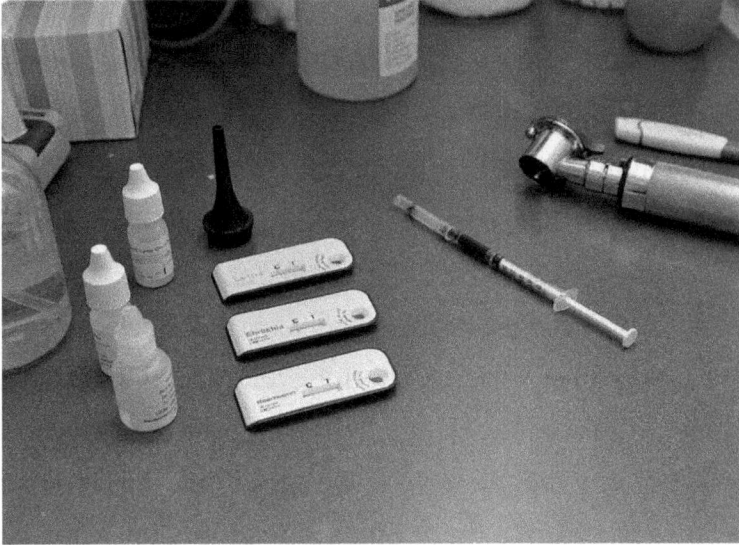

The diagnosis of Lyme disease is clinical. This means that while there is no definitive test to screen for the presence of Lyme disease, diagnosis is made based on an expert's evaluation of the results of various tests, the signs and symptoms you experience, and your medical history. It is always useful, therefore, to seek the help of a medical professional who has had some experience in dealing with Lyme disease.

## Diagnosing Lyme Disease

Lyme disease is not an easy disease to identify. Although the classic bull's eye rash (also called the Erythma migrans or EM) could be considered conclusive - this only happens less than 50% of the time. Many patients will only have a red papule at the tick bite without the characteristic bull's eye appearance, and others will not experience any rash at all. And because of the small size of the ticks and their painless bite, some might not even realize that they have been bitten by a tick at all. In the absence of the trademark EM or any telltale rash, one might think that they are simply suffering from a flu or other type of illness. Misdiagnosis is common, especially since the symptoms of Lyme disease bear striking similarity to other diseases such as MS, Chrohn's disease, Alzheimer's, Lups, or other psychiatric disorders.

That said, a clinical diagnosis of Lyme disease can be made based on a combination of the following factors:

### 1. Signs and symptoms

A person will seek the help of a medical practitioner once they feel that something is wrong. The various symptoms that a person may feel initially are varied, and the absence of some of the symptoms listed below does not necessarily exclude a diagnosis of Lyme disease. People's physiological reaction to the presence of the bacterium Borrelia burgdorferi are not always the same. But some of the most common signs that a person may feel, indicating a general sense of unwell-ness, can include:

- Becoming tired more easily
- Cramped and sore muscles
- Sensitivity to light
- Fever
- Headache
- A weird rash on the body that may or may not resemble a bull's eye mark

## 2. Medical history, and the possibility of exposure to infected carrier ticks

Your doctor will also be asking you your medical history. It is always possible that what you are experiencing may be the result of another disease or illness, and not Lyme disease. Just as it is possible to misdiagnose Lyme disease as something else, a misdiagnosed condition of Lyme disease will make it that much difficult for you to get better if you are not given appropriate treatment.

In asking about your medical history, the doctor will also need to consider the possibility of your having been exposed to infected ticks.  Thus, the following questions may be asked:

- Has anyone in your family or in your neighborhood recently been diagnosed with Lyme disease?  Or has anyone else been experiencing the same symptoms you are experiencing?
- Have you recently taken a trip to areas or regions with known tick infections?
- How often do you go outdoors?  When was the last time you have been outdoors?  Where was this, and was the terrain grassy, humid and rich with small animal wildlife?
- What steps or measures have you taken to protect yourself from insect bites?
- Did you wash and check yourself, your gear, and your clothes immediately after coming home?
- Were you accompanied by another family member, or a pet, and did you also check them for possible ticks?

## 3. Laboratory blood tests

It should be stated right at the beginning that blood tests are not conclusive in testing for Lyme disease. False negative results are common. This is because the more common tests administered in possible cases of Lyme disease do not test directly for the bacteria or for Lyme disease, but instead measure the body's antibody response to an infection. Antibody tests measure a body's response to bacterial infection, including the levels of antibody production.

### The two-tiered approach

The two most common antibody tests for Lyme disease are the ELISA test and a Western blot test. It should be noted that the CDC recommends a two-tier testing - an ELISA test to screen for Lyme disease, and then confirmation with a Western blot test. But even so, this two-tiered testing system can still miss roughly up to 54% of Lyme disease cases.

### ELISA test (Enzyme-linked immunosorbent assay)

The ELISA test works by measuring the body's production of antibodies to viruses or infectious bacteria like the Borrelia burgdorferi. As stated in a previous chapter, the spirochete of Lyme disease is quite adept in hiding from the body's immune system, and so even as the body mounts an immunological response, a person might not produce enough levels of antibodies or neutrophils to register on the ELISA scale, thus creating a false positive result.

But while not conclusive enough to be used as the sole basis for a diagnosis, a positive result in the ELISA test, coupled with the EM or the bull's eye rash, can be considered sufficient for a diagnosis of Lyme disease.

### Western blot test

The Western blot test is usually done to confirm a positive result in the ELISA test, and is the second and more specific phase to the prescribed two-tiered approach in testing for Lyme disease. But because of its greater specificity, there are some physicians who skip the ELISA test altogether and go straight to the Western blot test.

This test works by detecting antibodies to several proteins of Borrelia burgdorferi. Electricity is used to separate protein antigens into bands, and the results are compared to patterns of known cases of Lyme disease. If there are the right number of bands, and in the right places, then the result is positive. But it should be noted that the interpretation of the results can vary between different laboratories, and so what may be considered positive by some may be considered negative by others.

Again, this just goes to show that Lyme disease is not easy to diagnose, and so clinical diagnosis should be based on more than one of the factors listed above.

*Other tests*

There are other tests being used to diagnose Lyme disease, and these seek to detect the infectious bacteria Borrelia burgdorferi directly, not just the body's immune response. Even so, various factors - as shall be noted below - can serve to negate the results of each test, and so none of them can still be considered conclusive.

These tests include the following:

Polymerase chain reaction (PCR)

The PCR works by multiplying a key portion of the DNA from the Lyme bacteria so that it can be detected. But while highly accurate when the specified DNA is detected, accuracy is negated by the sparse nature of the bacteria, which may not even be present in the tested samples. Many false negative results may still be possible.

Antigen tests

Antigen tests seek out specific and unique Lyme proteins in fluids such as in blood or urine, but the results of this type of testing are still considered questionable.

### Culture testing

Considered the "gold standard" in evaluation of infections, culture testing works by taking blood or other fluid samples from a patient, and attempting the growth of Lyme spirochetes in a special medium.

The difficulty is that culture can take weeks, and it is rarely positive once the infection has grown beyond the stage of erythema migrans. Positive results may be produced during the EM stage, but there is usually a low yield for the late or disseminated stage of Lyme disease.

In addition, this is considered a new test and while available commercially to patients, they may still require further validation in other studies.

# Chapter Five: Treatment Options for Lyme Disease

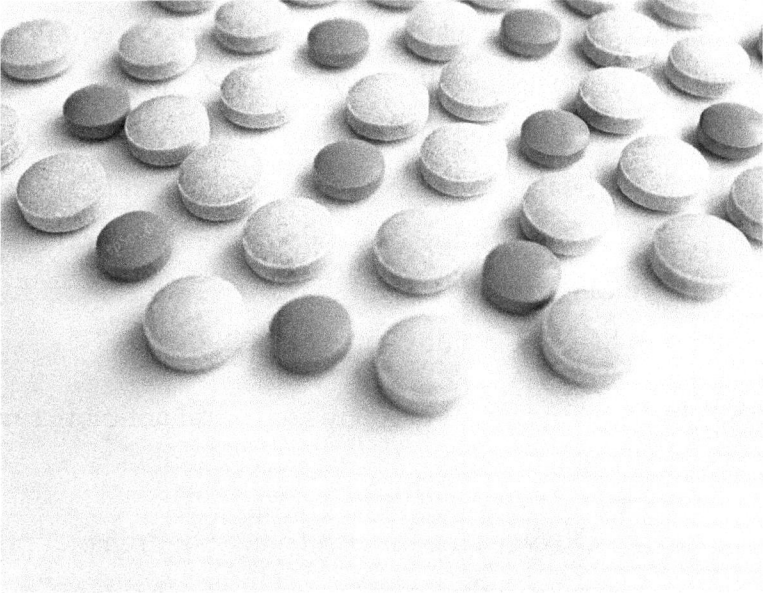

The best treatment, they say, is always prevention. But while prevention of Lyme disease is mostly centered upon reducing the risk of being bitten by infected ticks (see Chapter Two), even the most cautious person can sometimes fall prey to the bite of the Ixodes tick. In this chapter, we will look at the current treatment options available for those who have been diagnosed with Lyme disease.

*Antiobiotics for Lyme Disease*

Most experts agree that Lyme disease is best treated in its early stages, and the standard treatment involves oral antibiotics, a full course of which can last from 14 to 21 days, though some courses of 10 to 14 days can be equally effective. It is generally recommended, however, that a person should finish the full course of the antibiotics even if he or she begins to feel better. Lyme disease is, after all, notorious for avoiding detection, and finishing the prescribed full course of antibiotics would ensure that all foreign bacteria in your system are killed.

In the early stages of the disease, oral antibiotics may prescribed, including:

- Doxycycline for adults and children older than 8 years old
- Cefuroxime and Amoxicillin for adults, younger children, and women who are nursing or breast-feeding

Late stage or more severe cases of Lyme disease can be treated with intravenous antibiotics. This can be done for a period of 14 to 21 days. But while treatment can help to eliminate infection, the symptoms in late-stage Lyme disease may be slower to improve.

Other possible treatments for more severe cases of Lyme disease include intramuscular treatment, and pulse and combination therapy. In intramuscular treatment, the antibiotics are injected intramuscularly. This is particularly helpful for those who cannot tolerate oral antibiotics. Pulse and combination therapy, on the other hand, involve a careful combination of antibiotic treatments to coincide with symptom flare-ups.

This last option, while relatively new, is particularly interesting for the more severe cases of Lyme disease because while there is no clear consensus on the best treatment, recent studies in Canada have shown that a single course of antibiotics may not be sufficient for treating cases which have been undiagnosed and untreated for several months. This is because co-infections can occur, which can result in a more complicated case of Lyme disease.

This means that while a single course of oral antibiotics may be prescribed for early stage Lyme disease, if this course of treatment is insufficient, additional antibiotics, or even intravenous medication, may be prescribed. This is important because effective treatment of Lyme disease in its earlier stages yields the best patient outcome.

One possible side-effect to antibiotic treatment, however, is a resulting skin sensitivity to sunlight. Prolonged sun exposure is therefore not recommended until after treatment has been finished.

## *Alternative Treatments*

If you are looking to explore alternative and more holistic treatments for Lyme disease, please remember to exercise due care and caution. It is always best to do so with the approval of your medical practitioner. In fact, you might begin your exploration of alternative healing therapies by asking your doctor for any recommendations or referrals he may have. You don't want to create a conflict between different treatment options you may be taking, and it is never wise to discontinue active medical treatment.

Be discerning, selective and cautious in choosing alternative therapists or practitioners. Try to select those who are duly registered with appropriate governing bodies that regulate their practice to a certain extent. And most of all, since many alternative therapies are natural and holistic in their approach, be particularly wary of invasive alternative therapies such as injections. The Food and Drug Administration (FDA) has warned against an injectable compound sometimes used by alternative medicine practitioners to treat Lyme disease, because this might contain bismacine, a substance that can cause bismuth poisoning and which may lead to heart and kidney failure.

But healing is certainly a holistic process, and some might benefit greatly from taking alternative therapies or other preventive measures which, if they do not "cure" Lyme disease directly, may still benefit us by improving our overall quality of life and our outlook on our health, well being, and disease.

Some of the alternative ways by which a person can manage or prevent Lyme disease include:

### 1. Rest and stress management

Stress is the disease of modern times, it has been said by some; and it has certainly been the root of many health imbalances. Getting enough rest and proactively managing the constant stress that we go through daily can go a long way in boosting our immune system, thus reducing the chance for us to get sick.

More importantly, stress itself can serve as a trigger for inflammation and may even cause hormonal imbalances that can provide the Lyme bacteria optimal conditions in which to thrive. And since Lyme disease can cause severe fatigue and low energy in some people, enough rest and sleep is certainly necessary for effective healing and recuperation.

### 2. Improve cellular functions using supplements

Lyme disease can wreak havoc with our cellular health and functions, and this can result in vitamin deficiencies which may also compromise our immune system. Consult with your doctor and be tested for any deficiencies which you may have, and take the appropriate supplements, or adjust your diet and lifestyle accordingly to take in more of natural sources of vitamins and minerals.

### 3. Exercise

Moderate and regular exercise can strengthen one's muscles and overall muskoskeletal system, and this can also increase the oxygen levels in the blood which may help fight bacteria. Be sure to exercise moderately and within your limits, as Lyme disease can cause excessive fatigue and arthritic conditions.

### 4. Eat healthy

Consult with a nutrionist to maximize the benefits of a healthy diet. Aside from boosting your immunity, you can help speed your healing process by choosing anti-inflammatory and high-antioxidant foods. You can eat to address your specific nutrient deficiencies, reduce the foods that are harmful to your health, and naturally raise your immune system.

Some recommended foods for Lyme disease also include: bone broth, probiotic-rich foods such as yogurt to increase our store of good bacteria, leafy greens, cleansing tea, and lots of water.

5.  **Clean your surroundings to minimize the possibility of tick infections**

In line with preventive measures, you might wish to clean your house and yard regularly in order to reduce the possibility of tick infestations, as well as other parasitic infections. This is particularly true for those living in areas with known cases of Lyme disease infections, or those who are near woody or grassy areas. You can also use approved insecticides or pesticides to kill those that are already in your area, or you may bring in an exterminator and get the job done professionally.

Please exercise due caution in making use of pesticides or any poisonous or toxic chemicals. Observe all directions properly and be sure to wash your hands thoroughly after spraying or handling these substances. Minimize any exposure risks to yourself and your family and pets either through inhalation or ingesting.

And while you're at it, you might also want to give the family pet a thorough bath and examination to make sure that they are also tick- and parasite-free.

### 6. Acupuncture

There are those who claim great relief from Lyme disease symptoms with acupuncture treatments. Traditionally, acupuncture has been used alongside Chinese herbal medicines to cure or treat infectious diseases. More recent studies have also shown that acupuncture can provide Lyme disease patients with relief from symptoms such as joint pain and chronic fatigue.

Acupuncture is a form of traditional Chinese medicine that makes use of needles inserted into specific points, and is commonly used for pain relief though it has also been used as a treatment for a variety of other conditions.

There are regulatory bodies governing acupuncturists in countries such as the United States, the UK, Australia and Canada. The World Health Organization has recommended that a license or certification only be given to a physician after receiving at least 200 hours of specialized training, and 2,500 hours for non-physicians. Specific licensing requirements can vary between states, but the needles that are used in acupuncture are regulated by the FDA.

# Chapter Six: Controversies Surrounding Lyme Disease

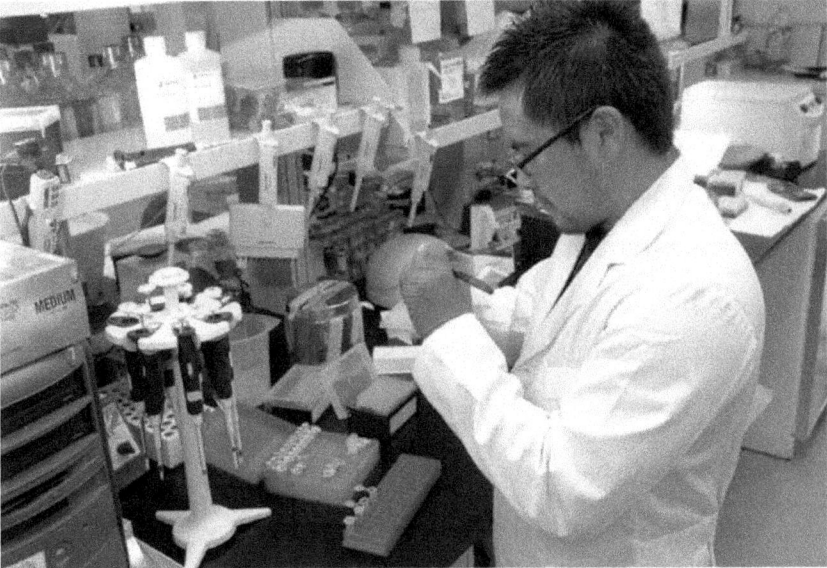

Lyme disease seems to be a pretty controversial disease, in more ways than one. Aside from the alleged source or origin of the bacteria Borrelia, which conspiracy theorists claim were developed by the government as a form of biological weapon that was released accidentally from Plum Island (see Chapter 1: History of Lyme Disease), rife controversy has also clouded two aspects of Lyme disease: the vaccine to prevent Lyme disease, and the existence or non-existence of Chronic Lyme disease.

*Vaccines*

A Lyme disease vaccine called LYMERix was once offered to the public, and studies have shown that it offers effective protection against the Lyme bacteria. But it was pulled out of the market by its manufacturer SmithKline Beecham (now GlaxoSmithKline) in 2002, citing insufficient consumer demand. The fact of it was that the vaccine was forced out of the market by lawsuits and the ensuing notoriety due to alleged adverse reactions among those who had received the vaccine. This, despite no scientific finding of a direct link between the vaccine and the claimed adverse effects.

This vaccine worked by stimulating antibodies that would attack the Lyme bacteria even while it was still in the tick's gut, as it fed on the human host, thereby killing the spirochete before it ever entered the host's body. Three doses of this vaccine resulted in about a 78% level of protection against the contraction of Lyme disease, and a 100% level of protecion against asymptomatic cases. So why is it no longer available?

Several factors contributed to the public outcry against this vaccine. First of all, it was only given permissive recommendation after having been licensed. With permissive licensing, it was not considered routinely recommended to everyone of a particular age group who did not have a contraindication to the vaccine - much as we do with our regular vaccines. The decision of administering the vaccine became a tricky affair then, as it was recommended to be used for "individuals between 15 and 70 years old living or working in areas with high rates of Lyme disease." This standard was potentially confusing and subject to varying interpretation, baffling both the populace and the administering doctors. And because it only had permissive recommendations, it was not considered covered by the National Vaccine Injury Compensation Program (NVICP).

Secondly, post-licensure monitoring brought in reports of adverse reactions as a result of the vaccine such as headaches, arthritis, and some alleged side-effects that were potentially life-threatening. But even as studies were being conducted to determine the causal link between the vaccine and the side-effects, heavy media coverage, anti-Lyme vaccine groups, and various lawsuits had all but forced the vaccine out of the market. The manufacturer then decided to withdraw the vaccine from the market and stop production in 2002.

The clincher is that the result of the studies showed no causal link between the vaccine and the reported side-effects. That is, the data showed no difference in the incidence of chronic arthritis between those who received the vaccine and those who did not. To put it another way, the data did not support findings that the reported adverse effects occurred at a higher rate than that expected among the population regardless of Lyme vaccination.

The result is that while a vaccine for Lyme disease may be available for our furry best friends, no such vaccine is available for humans.

## Chronic Lyme Disease

The controversy around Chronic Lyme disease lies in the fact that the very existence of this condition is being put into question. Experts claim that antibiotics work effectively to combat the bacterial infection in our bodies, and any lingering symptoms that a person may feel is due to what has been called "post-treatment Lyme disease syndrome (PTLDS)." It is quite likely that the lingering symptoms are caused by the prevalent damage triggered by the bacteria in the body such as auto-immune disorders, but not by the bacteria itself. According to the CDC, approximately 10 - 20% of Lyme disease patients can still experience various symptoms even after a full course of successful antibiotic treatments.

The controversy comes in due to the disagreement of a second group that claim that the condition is caused by lingering bacterial infection, thereby necessitating long-term antibiotic treatment that could go on for months or even years. If symptoms return after months or years, it is just possible that it has been caused by a recurrent infection, necessitating another course of antibiotics. But those who claim that there is no such thing as Chronic Lyme disease state that long-term antibiotic treatments are not really necessary, or even effective, and may serve nothing more than to give the patients a placebo effect. If there are recurring symptoms of an infection, it is just possible that it was caused by a new infection - another tick bite, or another tick-borne infection.

The difficulty is that diagnosis of everything related to Lyme disease and the spirochete Borrelia burgdorferi is clinical - and that includes Chronic Lyme disease. But while experts will not disagree that there are symptoms, identifying the cause and the course of treatment becomes problematic. These days, though, and despite the raging controversy, PTLDS is often simply referred to interchangeably as Chronic Lyme Disease. If the cause is a lingering bacterial infection, then perhaps long-term antibiotic treatments may be helpful, but authorities have already warned against their possible harmful and even dangerous effects. But on the other side of the coin, advocates for the recognition of Chronic Lyme disease are pushing for the acknowledgement of this disease, as well as insurance coverage for what they consider long-term antibiotic therapy.

Without further and conclusive research and study, however, there is still no scientific basis to prove or disprove either stand.

# Chapter Seven: The Future of Research Into Lyme Disease

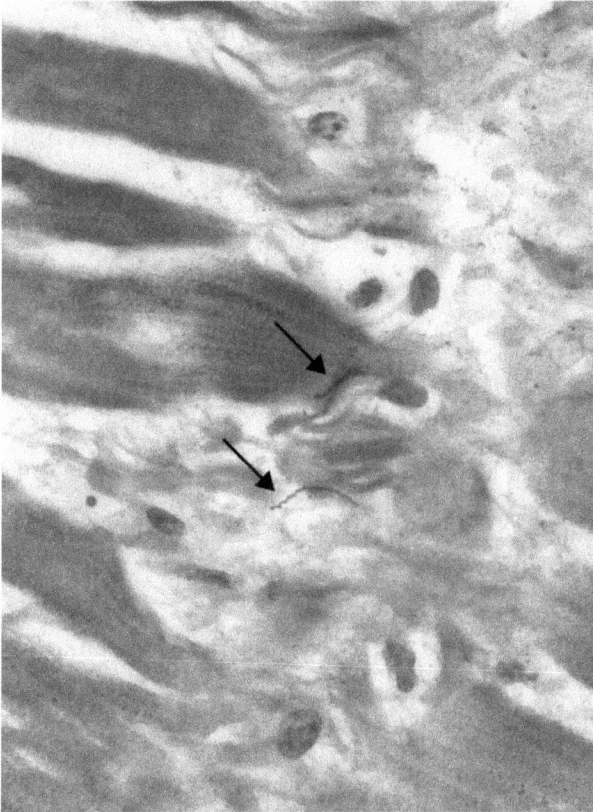

For such a prevalent disease, we still know relatively little about Lyme disease - so much so that large gaps in our knowledge still exist in terms of diagnosis and treatment options. And yet it is estimated that Lyme disease now afflicts more than 300,000 people each year in the United States alone, making it one of the most common infectious diseases in the world.

The National Institute of Allergy and Infectious Diseases (NIAID) of the NIH released a document last 2015, presenting the directions in which current and ongoing research efforts are going. These research efforts are centered around studies on:

- Vectors of the Disease
- Pathogenesis
- Persistence of Infection
- Diagnostic Testing
- Vaccines
- Autoimmunity and Lyme Disease

But the worldwide prevalence of Lyme disease has inspired research and study efforts in various laboratories in schools and hospitals all over the world, and the efforts lie along the same lines, including more effective treatments - mainly because the gap of our medical and scientific knowledge about Lyme disease and its variants are the same the world over.

In the meantime, spreading awareness about Lyme disease: what it is, how it is treated, and the ways and means of preventing or minimizing risks of exposure, should be a priority - not only among lay people, but also among medical staff and personnel. Not only can it help people avoid contracting the causal bacteria in the first place, but early diagnosis and treatment offers the best outlook for patients who contract the infection.

## Lyme FAQs

To sum up, here are a few quick facts about Lyme disease:

- Every year, about 300,000 cases of Lyme disease are reported in the U.S., but the CDC states that the actual number may actually be ten times higher.
- It takes 36 to 48 hours for an infected tick to transmit Lyme disease to a host, so immediately taking a bath and cleaning up your gear after having been outdoors can go a long way to preventing infection.
- The Lyme disease vaccine was discontinued in 2002. There are currently no Lyme vaccines available for humans.

- The most common and tell-tale symptom of Lyme disease is a rash that looks like a bull's eye. But less than 50% of those with Lyme disease will actually have this bull's eye rash.
- Diagnosis of Lyme disease is clinical.
- The symptoms of Lyme disease is similar to many other diseases, so misdiagnosis is quite common.
- A tick-bite is not easy to detect, and many patients who contract Lyme disease do not even recall being bitten.
- There is no test to show to eradication of the bacteria, or to show that a patient has been cured. Up to 40% experience long-term health problems, and this has been referred to interchangeably as Chronic Lyme Disease or Post-treatment Lyme Disease Syndrome (PTLDS).

# Index

## P

## R

## S

## T

## V

## W

# Photo References

Page 1 Photo by Oregon State University via Wikimedia Commons.
<https://commons.wikimedia.org/wiki/File:Tick_in_amber_c arrying_spirochetes.jpg>

Page 7 Photo by the CDC via the Public Health Image Library (PHIL).
<http://phil.cdc.gov/phil/details.asp?pid=3809>

Page 17 Photo by the CDC via the Public Health Image Library (PHIL).
http://phil.cdc.gov/Phil/details.asp?pid=14473

Page 27 Photo by the CDC via Wikimedia Commons.
<https://commons.wikimedia.org/wiki/File:Borrelia_burgdor feri-cropped.jpg>

Page 37 Photo by Airman 1st Class William Johnson via Wikimedia Commons.
<https://commons.wikimedia.org/wiki/File:Dover_Air_Force _Base_Veterinarian_Treatment_Facility_150227-F-PT194-016.jpg>

Page 45 Photo by epSos.de via Wikimedia Commons.
<https://commons.wikimedia.org/wiki/File:Medical_Drugs_f or_Pharmacy_Health_Shop_of_Medicine.png>

Page 55 Photo by National Institutes of Health via Wikimedia Commons. <https://commons.wikimedia.org/wiki/File:Medical_Laboratory_Scientist_US_NIH.jpg>

Page 61 Photo by Sherif Zaki, M.D. Ph.D. via CDC-PHIL. <http://phil.cdc.gov/Phil/details.asp?pid=19416>

# References

"5 Top Myths About Lyme Disease." Richard I. Horowitz. <http://bottomlineinc.com/5-top-myths-about-lyme-disease/>

"6 Lyme Disease Myths Debunked." Katie Moisse. <http://abcnews.go.com/Health/lyme-disease-myths-debunked/story?id=20010794#5>

"10 Essential Facts About Lyme Disease." Allison Pohle. <http://www.everydayhealth.com/news/10-essential-facts-about-lyme-disease/>

"10 Important Ways to Avoid Summer Tick Bites." Tia Ghose. <http://www.livescience.com/46160-how-to-avoid-tick-bites.html>

"10 Top Myths About Lyme Disease." Global Lyme Alliance. <http://www.lymeresearchalliance.org/index_10_myths.html>

"A History of Lyme Disease, Symptoms, Diagnosis, Treatment, and Prevention." NIH: National Institute of Allergy and Infectious Diseases. <https://www.niaid.nih.gov/topics/lymedisease/Pages/History.aspx>

"About Lyme Disease." lymedisease.org.
   <https://www.lymedisease.org/lyme-basics/lyme-
   disease/about-lyme/>

"Acupuncture." Wikipedia.
   <https://en.wikipedia.org/wiki/Acupuncture>

"Acupuncture for healing Lyme." LDRD. <http://www.lyme-
   disease-research-
   database.com/lyme_disease_blog_files/acupuncture-for-
   healing-lyme.html>

"Chronic Lyme Disease Myth - Reviewing the Evidence."
   The Original Skeptical Raptor.
   <http://www.skepticalraptor.com/skepticalraptorblog.ph
   p/chronic-lyme-disease-myth-reviewing-the-evidence/>

"Current Efforts in Lyme Disease Research, 2015." NIAID.
   <https://www.niaid.nih.gov/topics/lymeDisease/Docume
   nts/NIAIDLymereport2015.pdf>

"Current Studies in Progress." Lyme and Tick-Borne
   Diseases Research Center. <http://www.columbia-
   lyme.org/research/cr_research.html>

"Diagnosis and Testing." CDC.
   <http://www.cdc.gov/lyme/diagnosistesting/>

"ILADS About Lyme." International Lyme and Associated Diseases Society. <http://www.ilads.org/lyme/lyme-quickfacts.php>

"ELISA." MedlinePlus. <https://www.nlm.nih.gov/medlineplus/ency/article/003332.htm>

"FAQ: Infection." Lyme Disease Action. <http://www.lymediseaseaction.org.uk/about-lyme/faq/>

"Glossary." Lyme Disease Action. <http://www.lymediseaseaction.org.uk/resources/glossary/>

"Glossary." Tick Talk Ireland. <http://www.ticktalkireland.org/glossary.html>

"Glossary for Lyme disease." rightdiagnosis.com. <http://www.rightdiagnosis.com/l/lyme_disease/glossary.htm>

"History of Lyme Disease." Bay Area Lyme Foundation. <http://www.bayarealyme.org/about-lyme/history-lyme-disease/>

"History of Lyme Disease." Medscape. <http://www.medscape.com/viewarticle/807929_2>

"How To Cure Lyme Disease, And Virtually Any Other Bacterial Infection, Naturally." Michael Edwards. <http://www.organiclifestylemagazine.com/issue/15-how-to-cure-lyme-disease-and-virtually-any-other-bacterial-infection-naturally>

"Ixodes." Wikipedia. <https://en.wikipedia.org/wiki/Ixodes>

"Ixodidae." Wikipedia. <https://en.wikipedia.org/wiki/Ixodidae>

"Laboratory Tests." Columbia University Medical Center: Lyme and Tick-Borne Diseases Research Center. <http://www.columbia-lyme.org/patients/ld_lab_test.html>

"Lyme Diagnosis." Canadian Lyme Disease Foundation. <http://canlyme.com/just-diagnosed/>

"Lyme Disease." The Healthline Editorial Team. <http://www.healthline.com/health/lyme-disease>

"Lyme Disease." John O. Meyerhoff, MD and Herbert S Diamond, MD. <http://emedicine.medscape.com/article/330178-overview>

"Lyme Disease: Treatment and Drugs." Mayo Clinic Staff.
    <http://www.mayoclinic.org/diseases-conditions/lyme-
    disease/basics/treatment/con-20019701>

"Lyme Disease." Merck Manual.
    <http://www.merckmanuals.com/professional/infectious-
    diseases/spirochetes/lyme-disease>

"Lyme Disease." NHS Choices.
    <http://www.nhs.uk/conditions/Lyme-
    disease/Pages/Introduction.aspx>

"Lyme Disease." Wikipedia.
    <https://en.wikipedia.org/wiki/Lyme_disease>

"Lyme disease controversy." Wikipedia.
    <https://en.wikipedia.org/wiki/Lyme_disease_controvers
    y>

"Lyme Disease Diagnosis. lymedisease.org.
    <https://www.lymedisease.org/lyme-basics/lyme-
    disease/diagnosis/>

"Lyme Disease Glossary of Terms." emedicinehealth.com.
    <http://www.emedicinehealth.com/lyme_disease/glossar
    y_em.htm>

"Lyme disease is spreading faster than ever and humans are
    partly to blame." Gwynn Guilford.

<http://qz.com/441583/lyme-disease-is-spreading-faster-than-ever-and-humans-are-partly-to-blame/>

"Lyme Disease on Plum Island: Fringe Conspiracy Theory or Government Cover-up?" Smaranda Dumitru. <https://sites.newpaltz.edu/ticktalk/social-attitudes/story-by-smaranda-dumitru/>

"Lyme Disease Pathology." LymeDiseaseGuide.org. <http://lymediseaseguide.org/lyme-disease-pathology>

"Lyme Disease Treatment." lymedisease.org. <https://www.lymedisease.org/lyme-basics/lyme-disease/treatment/>

"Lyme Disease Treatment (Natural vs. Conventional) + Prevention Tips." Dr. Axe. <https://draxe.com/natural-strategies-to-cure-lyme-disease/>

"Lyme Disease Vaccine." CDC. <http://www.cdc.gov/lyme/prev/vaccine.html>

"Lyme Myths." Canadian Lyme Disease Foundation. <http://canlyme.com/lyme-basics/lyme-myths/>

"Myths of Lyme Disease." Bay Area Lyme Foundation. <http://www.bayarealyme.org/about-lyme/myths/>

"Pathogenesis of Lyme Disease and Gene Expression in Borrelia burgdorferi." MicrobeWiki.

<https://microbewiki.kenyon.edu/index.php/Pathogenesis_of_Lyme_Disease_and_Gene_Expression_in_Borrelia_burgdorferi>

"Post-Treatment Lyme Disease Syndrome." CDC. <http://www.cdc.gov/lyme/postlds/>

"Prevent Tick Bites While Enjoying the Outdoors." Robert Preidt. <http://www.webmd.com/skin-problems-and-treatments/news/20140413/prevent-tick-bites-while-enjoying-the-outdoors>

"Preventing Tick Bites." CDC. <http://www.cdc.gov/ticks/avoid/on_people.html>

"Stop Ticks." CDC. <http://www.cdc.gov/features/stopticks/>

"Suspect Lyme?" Canadian Lyme Disease Foundation. <http://canlyme.com/just-diagnosed/next-steps/>

"Testing." Canadian Lyme Disease Foundation. <http://canlyme.com/just-diagnosed/testing/>

"Tests and Diagnosis." Mayoclinic.org. <http://www.mayoclinic.org/diseases-conditions/lyme-disease/basics/tests-diagnosis/con-20019701>

"The History of the Lyme Disease Vaccine." The History of Vaccines.

<http://www.historyofvaccines.org/content/articles/histor
y-lyme-disease-vaccine>

"The Top Natural Treatments for Lyme Disease." Leah
Zerbe. <http://www.rodalewellness.com/health/lyme-
disease-treatment>

"There's An Effective Vaccine For Lyme Disease - But You
Can't Get It, Thanks To Anti-Vaxxers." Justine Alford.
<http://www.iflscience.com/health-and-medicine/thanks-
anti-vaxxers-only-licensed-lyme-disease-vaccine-was-
withdrawn/>

"Tick." Wikipedia. <https://en.wikipedia.org/wiki/Tick>

"Tick Removal." CDC.
<http://www.cdc.gov/ticks/removing_a_tick.html>

"Transmission." Canadian Lyme Disease Foundation.
<http://canlyme.com/lyme-prevention/transmission/>

"Treatment." Canadian Lyme Disease Foundation.
<http://canlyme.com/just-diagnosed/treatment/>

"What is Lyme Disease? New Findings Deepen the Mystery."
Jarret Liotta, for National Geographic.
<http://news.nationalgeographic.com/news/2014/02/1402
28-lyme-disease-borrelia-burgdorferi-deer-tick-science/>

"What is the history of Lyme disease?" William C. Shiel, Jr. MD, FACP, FACR. <http://www.medicinenet.com/lyme_disease/page3.htm>

"What You Should Know About Chronic Lyme Disease." Hallie Levine. <http://news.health.com/2015/01/23/yolanda-foster-chronic-lyme-disease/>

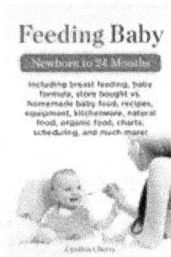

Feeding Baby
Cynthia Cherry
978-1941070000

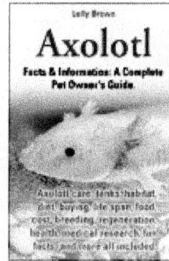

Axolotl
Lolly Brown
978-0989658430

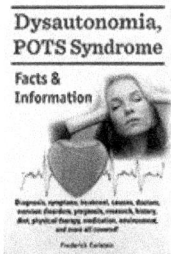

Dysautonomia, POTS
Syndrome
Frederick Earlstein
978-0989658485

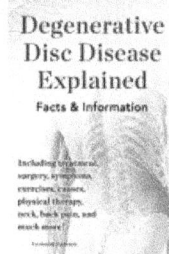

Degenerative Disc
Disease Explained
Frederick Earlstein
978-0989658485

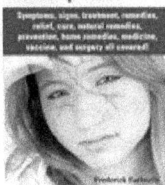

Sinusitis, Hay Fever,
Allergic Rhinitis Explained
Frederick Earlstein
978-1941070024

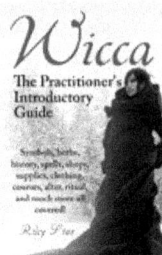

Wicca
Riley Star
978-1941070130

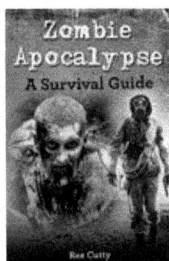

Zombie Apocalypse
Rex Cutty
978-1941070154

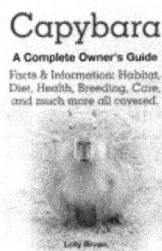

Capybara
Lolly Brown
978-1941070062

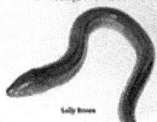

Eels As Pets
Lolly Brown
978-1941070167

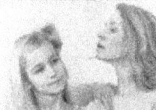

Scabies and Lice Explained
Frederick Earlstein
978-1941070017

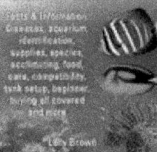

Saltwater Fish As Pets
Lolly Brown
978-0989658461

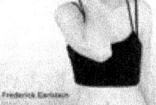

Torticollis Explained
Frederick Earlstein
978-1941070055

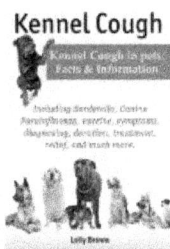

Kennel Cough
Lolly Brown
978-0989658409

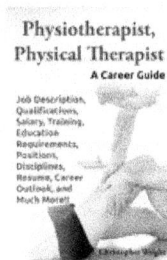

Physiotherapist, Physical
Therapist
Christopher Wright
978-0989658492

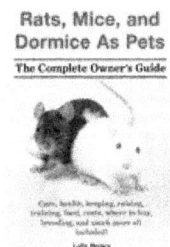

Rats, Mice, and Dormice
As Pets
Lolly Brown
978-1941070079

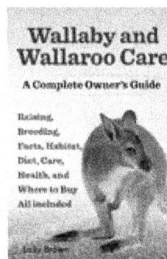

Wallaby and Wallaroo Care
Lolly Brown
978-1941070031

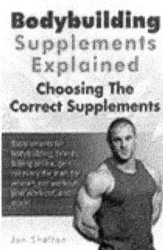

Bodybuilding Supplements
Explained
Jon Shelton
978-1941070239

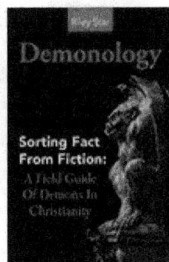

Demonology
Riley Star
978-19401070314

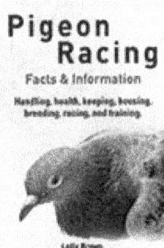

Pigeon Racing
Lolly Brown
978-1941070307

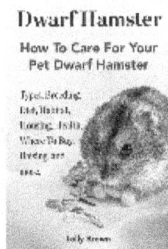

Dwarf Hamster
Lolly Brown
978-1941070390

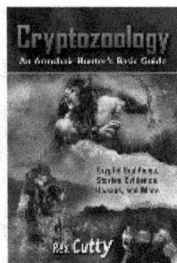

Cryptozoology
Rex Cutty
978-1941070406

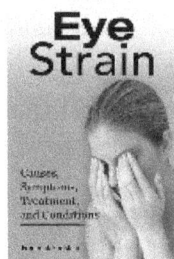

Eye Strain
Frederick Earlstein
978-1941070369

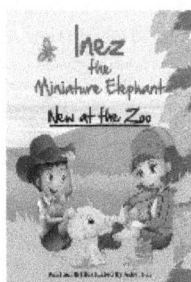

Inez The Miniature Elephant
Asher Ray
978-1941070353

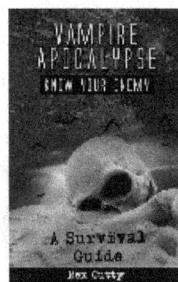

Vampire Apocalypse
Rex Cutty
978-1941070321

www.ingramcontent.com/pod-product-compliance
Lightning Source LLC
Chambersburg PA
CBHW060636210326
41520CB00010B/1620